Unlocking Wellness

Reversing Hypertension Naturally

Daniel C. Wright

Table of Contents

7. CHAPTER SEVEN: Case Studies and Success Stories on Hypertension Reversal

Conclusion

Introduction

Hypertension, commonly known as high blood pressure, is a prevalent health condition that affects millions of individuals worldwide. It occurs when the force of blood against the walls of the arteries is consistently too high, leading to potential complications such as heart disease, stroke, and kidney problems. While there are various medical approaches to managing hypertension, this book aims to provide a natural and holistic perspective on reversing this condition.

In this introductory chapter, we will explore the overview of hypertension and the importance of addressing it naturally. Hypertension is often referred to as the "silent killer" because it typically has no symptoms until it reaches advanced stages. Understanding the nature of hypertension, its causes, and risk factors is crucial in developing effective strategies to reverse it.

Conventional medical treatments for hypertension often involve medications to lower blood pressure and reduce the risk of complications. However, these medications may come with side effects and may not address the underlying causes of hypertension. This is where natural remedies and lifestyle modifications come into play.

The natural remedies section of this book will delve into the role of nutrition and diet in promoting healthy blood pressure levels. We will explore the benefits of herbal and supplemental therapies, as well as physical activity and exercise techniques specifically designed to lower blood pressure. Additionally, stress management and relaxation techniques will be discussed as effective ways to reduce hypertension.

Way of life changes assume an essential part in overseeing hypertension. Adopting a healthy lifestyle that includes managing weight, quitting smoking, moderating alcohol consumption, and improving sleep quality can significantly impact blood pressure levels.

Complementary and alternative therapies, such as acupuncture, traditional Chinese medicine, Ayurveda, and homeopathy, will also be explored as potential approaches to lower blood pressure naturally.

Prevention strategies will be emphasized throughout the book, highlighting the importance of regular check-ups, implementing dietary approaches, engaging in regular physical activity, and practicing stress reduction techniques. By adopting these strategies, individuals can reduce their risk of developing hypertension and maintain healthy blood pressure levels.

To illustrate the effectiveness of natural approaches, this book will include case studies and success stories of individuals who have successfully reversed hypertension. Their experiences will serve as inspiration and motivation for readers on their own journey towards lowering blood pressure naturally.

In conclusion, this book aims to provide a comprehensive guide on reversing hypertension in a natural way. By addressing the root causes, implementing natural remedies, making lifestyle modifications, and adopting prevention strategies, individuals can regain control over their blood pressure and improve their overall health. Let's embark on this journey together and discover the power of natural healing.

CHAPTER ONE
Understanding Hypertension

Hypertension, also known as high blood pressure, is a common medical condition that affects a significant portion of the population. It occurs when the force of blood against the walls of the arteries is consistently too high, putting strain on the cardiovascular system. Hypertension is often referred to as the "silent killer" because it typically has no symptoms until it reaches advanced stages.

To comprehend hypertension, it is essential to understand the idea of pulse and the job of cardiovascular framework. Circulatory strain is the power applied by circling blood against the walls of the veins. It is estimated utilizing two numbers: systolic tension (the larger number) and diastolic strain (the lower number. Systolic pressure represents the force when the heart contracts and pumps blood, while diastolic pressure represents the force when the heart is at rest between beats.

There are two kinds of hypertension: Essential (fundamental) hypertension and auxiliary hypertension. Essential hypertension is the most widely recognized type and has no recognizable reason. It is often associated with lifestyle factors such as poor diet, lack of exercise, stress, and obesity. Secondary hypertension, on the other hand, is caused by an underlying medical condition such as kidney disease, hormonal disorders, or certain medications.

Several risk factors contribute to the development of hypertension. These include age (risk increases with age), family history of hypertension, being overweight or obese, smoking, excessive alcohol consumption, a sedentary lifestyle, stress, and certain medical conditions such as diabetes and high cholesterol.

Hypertension can have serious wellbeing suggestions whenever left untreated. It puts strain on the heart, arteries, and other organs, increasing the risk of heart disease, stroke, kidney problems, and other complications. It is important to monitor blood pressure regularly and take steps to manage and lower it if necessary.

Treatment for hypertension typically involves a combination of lifestyle modifications and, in some cases, medication. Lifestyle modifications include adopting a healthy diet rich in fruits, vegetables, whole grains, and lean proteins, reducing sodium intake, engaging in regular physical activity, managing stress, quitting smoking, moderating alcohol consumption, and maintaining a healthy weight. Meds might be endorsed to bring down pulse in the event that way of life changes alone are not adequatent.

Understanding hypertension is the first step towards effectively managing and reversing this condition. By making positive lifestyle changes and working closely with healthcare professionals, individuals can take control of their blood pressure and reduce the risk of complications. Regular monitoring and adherence to treatment plans are crucial in maintaining optimal blood pressure levels and overall cardiovascular health.

CHAPTER TWO
Medical Approaches to Hypertension

Hypertension, generally known as high blood pressure, is a current health condition that affects millions of individualities worldwide. One of the primary medical approaches to hypertension is the use of antihypertensive specifics. These specifics works by relaxing blood vessels, reducing the volume of blood pressure, or dwindling the force of the heart condensation.

One of the primary medical approaches to hypertension is the use of antihypertensive medications. These medications work by relaxing blood vessels, reducing the volume of blood, or decreasing the force of the heart's contractions. There are several classes of antihypertensive medications, including diuretics, beta-blockers, ACE inhibitors, angiotensin receptor blockers (ARBs), and calcium channel blockers. The choice of medication depends on various factors, such as the patient's age, medical history, and other existing health conditions.

In addition to medications, lifestyle modifications play a crucial role in managing hypertension. These modifications include adopting a healthy diet, engaging in regular physical activity, limiting alcohol consumption, quitting smoking, and managing stress. A combination of medication and lifestyle changes is often recommended to achieve optimal blood pressure control.

For individuals with severe hypertension or those who do not respond well to medications, additional medical interventions may be necessary. One such intervention is renal denervation, a procedure that involves using radiofrequency energy to disrupt the nerves in the kidneys that contribute to high blood pressure. Renal denervation has shown promising results in reducing blood pressure in certain patients.

Another medical approach to hypertension is the use of implantable devices, such as baroreceptor activation therapy. This therapy involves implanting a small device near the carotid artery that stimulates the baroreceptors, which are responsible for regulating blood pressure. By activating these receptors, blood pressure can be lowered effectively.

It is important to note that hypertension management is a lifelong commitment. Regular monitoring of blood pressure is essential to ensure that it remains within the target range. This can be done at home using a blood pressure monitor or during regular check-ups with a healthcare provider.

In conclusion, the medical approaches to hypertension encompass a range of interventions, including medications, lifestyle modifications, renal denervation, and implantable devices. These approaches aim to lower blood pressure and reduce the risk of complications associated with hypertension. It is crucial for individuals with hypertension to work closely with their healthcare providers to develop a personalized treatment plan that suits their specific needs.

CHAPTER THREE
Natural Remedies for Hypertension

Hypertension, commonly known as high blood pressure, is a prevalent health condition that affects millions of individuals worldwide. While medical approaches are often necessary to manage hypertension effectively, there are also natural remedies that can help support blood pressure control. These natural remedies, when used in conjunction with medical treatment, may provide additional benefits.

One natural remedy for hypertension is adopting a healthy diet. The Dietary Approaches to Stop Hypertension (DASH) diet is often recommended for individuals with high blood pressure. This diet emphasizes consuming fruits, vegetables, whole grains, lean proteins, and low-fat dairy products while limiting sodium, saturated fats, and added sugars. The DASH diet has been shown to lower blood pressure and reduce the risk of heart disease.

Regular physical activity is another natural remedy that can help manage hypertension. Engaging in aerobic exercises, such as brisk walking, swimming, or cycling, for at least 150 minutes per week can help lower blood pressure. Physical activity helps strengthen the heart, improve blood circulation, and promote overall cardiovascular health.

Certain herbs and supplements have also been studied for their potential blood pressure-lowering effects. For example, garlic supplements have been shown to modestly reduce blood pressure in individuals with hypertension. Other herbs and supplements that may have a positive impact on blood pressure include hibiscus, fish oil, coenzyme Q10, and magnesium. However, it is important to consult with a healthcare provider before starting any new supplements, as they may interact with medications or have other side effects.

Stress management techniques, such as meditation, deep breathing exercises, and yoga, can also help lower blood pressure. Chronic stress can contribute to hypertension, so finding healthy ways to manage stress is crucial.

In addition to these natural remedies, it is important to maintain a healthy weight, limit alcohol consumption, and avoid smoking, as these factors can contribute to high blood pressure.

It is important to note that while natural remedies can be beneficial, they should not replace medical treatment for hypertension. It is essential to work closely with a healthcare provider to develop a comprehensive treatment plan that includes both medical approaches and natural remedies.

In conclusion, natural remedies can be used as complementary approaches to support blood pressure control in individuals with hypertension. Adopting a healthy diet, engaging in regular physical activity, managing stress, and considering certain herbs and supplements may provide additional benefits. However, it is important to consult with a healthcare provider before making any significant changes to your treatment plan.

CHAPTER FOUR
Lifestyle Modifications for Hypertension

Hypertension, also known as high blood pressure, is a common health condition that affects millions of people worldwide. While medical treatments are often necessary to manage hypertension effectively, lifestyle modifications can play a significant role in controlling blood pressure and reducing the risk of complications. Here are some key lifestyle changes that can help individuals with hypertension:

1. Adopting a Healthy Diet: Eating a balanced diet rich in fruits, vegetables, whole grains, lean proteins, and low-fat dairy products can have a positive impact on blood pressure. The Dietary Approaches to Stop Hypertension (DASH) diet is often recommended for individuals with high blood pressure, as it emphasizes reducing sodium intake and increasing potassium-rich foods.

2. Limiting Sodium Intake: Excessive salt consumption can contribute to high blood pressure. It is important to reduce the amount of salt added to meals and avoid processed foods that are high in sodium. Reading food labels and opting for low-sodium alternatives can help in managing salt intake.

3. Engaging in Regular Physical activity:

Regular exercise has numerous benefits for individuals with hypertension. Engaging in aerobic conditioning, similar as brisk walking, swimming, jogging, cycling, for at least 150 twinkles per week can help lower blood pressure. . Physical activity strengthens the heart, improves blood circulation, and promotes overall cardiovascular health.

4. Maintaining a Healthy Weight:

Being overweight or obese can increase the risk of hypertension. Losing excess weight through a combination of healthy eating and regular exercise can have a positive impact on blood pressure.

5. Limiting Alcohol Consumption:

inordinate alcohol consumption can raise blood pressure. It's recommended to limit alcohol input to moderate situations, which means up to one drink per day for women and up to two drinks per day for men.

6. Quitting Smoking: Smoking can contribute to high blood pressure and increase the risk of heart disease. Quitting smoking is essential for overall cardiovascular health and blood pressure control.

7. Managing Stress: Chronic stress can contribute to hypertension. Practicing stress management techniques, such as meditation, deep breathing exercises, yoga, or engaging in hobbies and activities that promote relaxation, can help lower blood pressure.

It is important to note that lifestyle modifications should not replace medical treatment for hypertension but should be used as complementary approaches. It is crucial to work closely with a healthcare provider to develop a comprehensive treatment plan that includes both medical approaches and lifestyle modifications.

In conclusion, lifestyle modifications are essential for managing hypertension effectively. Adopting a healthy diet, limiting sodium intake, engaging in regular physical activity, maintaining a healthy weight, limiting alcohol consumption, quitting smoking, and managing stress can all contribute to blood pressure control and overall cardiovascular health.

CHAPTER FIVE
Complementary and Alternative Therapies for Hypertension

Hypertension, commonly known as high blood pressure, is a prevalent health condition that requires medical intervention for effective management. However, some individuals with hypertension may also explore complementary and alternative therapies to support their treatment plan. While these therapies should not replace medical treatment, they can be used as adjunct approaches to promote overall well-being. Here are some complementary and alternative therapies that may be beneficial for individuals with hypertension:

1. Acupuncture: Acupuncture is an ancient Chinese practice that involves fitting thin needles into specific points on the body. It is believed to help balance the flow of energy and promote relaxation. Some studies have suggested that acupuncture may help lower blood pressure in individuals with hypertension.

2. Mind-body Techniques: Stress management techniques, such as meditation, deep breathing exercises, and yoga, can help reduce stress levels and promote relaxation. Chronic stress can contribute to hypertension, so incorporating these techniques into a daily routine can have a positive impact on blood pressure.

3. Massage Therapy: Massage therapy involves manipulating the body's soft tissues to promote relaxation and relieve muscle tension. It has been shown to help lower blood pressure and reduce anxiety and stress levels.

4. Herbal Remedies: Certain herbs, such as garlic, hibiscus, and olive leaf extract, have been studied for their potential blood pressure-lowering effects. However, it is important to consult with a healthcare provider before starting any herbal remedies, as they may interact with medications or have other side effects.

5. Biofeedback: Biofeedback is a technique that uses electronic devices to provide information about the body's physiological processes, such as heart rate and blood pressure. By learning to control these processes, individualities can potentially lower their blood pressure.

6. Dietary Supplements: Some individuals may consider taking dietary supplements, such as omega-3 fatty acids, coenzyme Q10, or magnesium, to support blood pressure control. However, it is important to consult with a healthcare provider before starting any new supplements, as they may interact with medications or have other side effects.

It is important to note that while complementary and alternative therapies may provide additional benefits, they should not replace medical treatment for hypertension. It is essential to work closely with a healthcare provider to develop a comprehensive treatment plan that includes both medical approaches and complementary therapies.

In conclusion, complementary and alternative therapies can be used as adjunct approaches to support the management of hypertension.

Acupuncture, mind-body techniques, massage therapy, herbal remedies, biofeedback, and dietary supplements may provide additional benefits. However, it is important to consult with a healthcare provider before incorporating these therapies into a treatment plan.

CHAPTER SIX

Prevention Strategies for Hypertension

Hypertension, commonly known as high blood pressure, is a prevalent medical condition that significantly increases the risk of heart disease, stroke, and other cardiovascular issues. The good news is that there are several effective prevention strategies that individuals can adopt to manage and lower their blood pressure levels, thereby reducing their risk of developing hypertension.

Healthy Diet: A balanced diet rich in fruits, vegetables, whole grains, lean proteins, and low-fat dairy products can contribute to lower blood pressure. Reducing sodium intake and avoiding processed foods high in salt is crucial, as excess sodium can lead to fluid retention and elevated blood pressure.

Regular Exercise: Engaging in regular physical activity can help maintain a healthy weight and improve cardiovascular health. Aim for at least 150 minutes of moderate-intensity aerobic exercise or 75 minutes of vigorous exercise each week, along with muscle-strengthening activities on two or more days.

Maintain a Healthy Weight: Maintaining a healthy weight range is essential in preventing hypertension. Excess body weight strains the cardiovascular system, increasing the risk of high blood pressure. Losing Indeed a small quantum of weight can have a positive impact on blood pressure situations.

Limit Alcohol and Caffeine: Limit Alcohol & Caffeine Excessive alcohol and caffeine consumption can raise blood pressure. Moderation is key; for alcohol, this means up to one drink per day for women and up to two drinks per day for men.

Manage Stress: Habitual Stress can contribute to high blood pressure. Practicing relaxation techniques such as deep breathing, meditation, yoga, or engaging in hobbies can help manage stress levels.

Quit Smoking: Smoking damages blood vessels and raises blood pressure.
towards preventing hypertension and improving overall cardiovascular health.

Regular Health Check-ups: Regular visits to a healthcare professional are important for monitoring blood pressure and overall health. Early detection and management of any blood pressure concerns can help prevent the progression of hypertension.

Limit Processed Foods: Processed and packaged foods often contain high levels of sodium, unhealthy fats, and sugars, all of which can contribute to high blood pressure. Reading nutrition labels and opting for fresh, whole foods is advisable.

By adopting a combination of these preventive strategies, individuals can significantly reduce their risk of developing hypertension and its associated health complications. It's important to remember that prevention is a lifelong commitment, and making small, sustainable changes to one's lifestyle can yield substantial benefits for long-term cardiovascular health.

CHAPTER SEVEN
Case Studies and Success Stories on Hypertension Reversal

Case studies and success stories focused on hypertension reversal highlight the remarkable potential of lifestyle modifications in combating this prevalent health issue. Hypertension, or high blood pressure, affects millions worldwide and is a major risk factor for cardiovascular diseases. While medication is commonly prescribed, these case studies underscore the effectiveness of alternative approaches in achieving long-lasting and sustainable results.

One such inspiring case study involves a middle-aged individual diagnosed with severe hypertension. Frustrated with the side effects of medication, they embarked on a comprehensive lifestyle overhaul. Through a combination of regular exercise, a balanced diet rich in whole foods, and stress-reduction techniques like meditation and yoga, they achieved significant blood pressure reduction over a span of six months. This success not only improved their health but also enhanced their overall quality of life.

Another noteworthy success story features a community-based initiative aimed at tackling hypertension. In a collaboration between healthcare professionals and local organizations, a holistic approach was taken. Public awareness campaigns educated residents about the risks of hypertension and the benefits of adopting healthier habits. Regular health check-ups, dietary workshops, and fitness classes were provided, resulting in a measurable decrease in hypertension rates within the community over the course of a year.

These case studies collectively underline the importance of a multi-faceted approach to hypertension reversal. Lifestyle modifications encompassing dietary improvements, physical activity, stress management, and community engagement can yield remarkable outcomes. Importantly, these success stories emphasize the potential for sustainable change – where individuals not only experience reduced blood pressure but also enjoy enhanced well-being on various levels.

In conclusion, the case studies and success stories centered around hypertension reversal serve as powerful testimonials to the efficacy of lifestyle changes in managing this health condition. They demonstrate that with determination, education, and comprehensive interventions, individuals and communities can overcome the challenges of hypertension, leading to healthier and happier lives. These stories provide valuable insights and inspiration for both healthcare professionals and those seeking alternative paths to better cardiovascular health.

Conclusion

In the realm of health and wellness, the stories of hypertension reversal through natural means offer a glimmer of hope and inspiration. These accounts reveal the incredible potential of our bodies to heal when we align ourselves with the rhythms of nature. As the world grapples with rising rates of high blood pressure and its associated risks, these tales remind us that there exists a path less traveled – one that involves embracing simple yet profound changes in our lifestyles.

The case studies and success stories discussed above exemplify the transformative power of holistic approaches. They show us that medication is not always the sole answer; rather, a harmonious integration of wholesome nutrition, physical activity, stress reduction, and community support can work wonders. These narratives underscore the importance of tapping into the innate wisdom of our bodies and making choices that align with our natural state of balance.

Through these stories, we witness individuals stepping into their own agency and becoming the architects of their health. Their journeys of hypertension reversal reflect a deeper connection with their bodies and environments, illustrating that nature offers a multitude of remedies for the ailments that afflict us. Whether it's the rejuvenating effect of nourishing foods, the vitality unlocked through mindful movement, or the peace found in cultivating inner stillness, these pathways pave the way for a renewed sense of well-being.

In the hustle and bustle of modern life, these tales serve as gentle reminders that our bodies are not separate from the natural world – they are an integral part of it. The successes recounted here are a celebration of the human spirit's resilience and adaptability, as well as a tribute to the healing potential of embracing nature's gifts.

As we navigate the complexities of health management, let us draw inspiration from these stories and consider the profound impact that a return to nature can have. By fostering a symbiotic relationship with our bodies and the environment, we can not only reverse hypertension but also foster a state of thriving vitality that resonates with the core essence of who we are.

www.ingramcontent.com/pod-product-compliance
Lightning Source LLC
Chambersburg PA
CBHW070744260726
48660CB00007B/2968